Fats

Fast Food Fat

By Cathy Wilson
Copyright © 2014

ISBN-13:
978-1505722079

ISBN-10:
1505722071

First Printing, 2014

Printed in the United States of America

Income Disclaimer

This book contains business strategies, marketing methods and other business advice that, regardless of my own results and experience, may not produce the same results (or any results) for you. I make absolutely no guarantee, expressed or implied, that by following the advice below you will make any money or improve current profits, as there are several factors and variables that come into play regarding any given business.

Primarily, results will depend on the nature of the product or business model, the conditions of the marketplace, the experience of the individual, and situations and elements that are beyond your control.
As with any business endeavor, you assume all risk related to investment and money based on your own discretion and at your own potential expense.

Liability Disclaimer

By reading this book, you assume all risks associated with using the advice given below, with a full understanding that you, solely, are responsible for anything that may occur as a result of putting this information into action in any way, and regardless of your interpretation of the advice.
You further agree that our company cannot be held responsible in any way for the success or failure of your business as a result of the information presented in this book. It is your responsibility to conduct your own due diligence regarding the safe and successful operation of your business if you intend to apply any of our information in any way to your business operations.

Terms of Use

You are given a non-transferable, "personal use" license to this book. You cannot distribute it or share it with other individuals.

Also, there are no resale rights or private label rights granted when purchasing this book. In other words, it's for your own personal use only.

Fats

Fast Food Fat

By Cathy Wilson

Table of Contents

Introduction

Here's a bit of the technical side of fat.

Medical News says a **Lipoprotein** is a medley of biochemical assembly containing proteins and fats, or lipids. These lipids are non-covalently or covalently hitched to proteins. Lipoproteins can come in the form of antigens, toxins, antigens, enzymes, structured proteins, or transporters.

Don't fret! This isn't a nightmare chemistry class, and don't forget this is an introductory book. So I'm not going to load you up with the scientific crap (I say that with a smile). But will acknowledge some of it is necessary when understanding fat and the role it plays in your health and wellness today.

The specific lipoproteins we're gonna zone in on a little are LDL or low-density lipoprotein, and HDL or high-density lipoprotein. Better known as bad and good cholesterol respectively, or fat in the blood, respectively.

DANGER ZONE FAT FACT - The worst of the worst in fat types is *synthetic* trans fat. I'll talk later about minute amounts of natural trans fat that are argued healthy by scientists.

These processed fake trans fats found in packaged cookies, cakes, pastries, and fast foods in particular, are deadly over time because they actively lower your good HDL cholesterol, and raise the naughty LDL cholesterol. This increases your risk for cardiovascular disease, stroke, and diabetes to start.

Understanding the good and bad of fat, how much you need, what foods to get it from, and how to better manage fat, helps you lose weight quickly, improve protective immune system function, increase energy, and stay healthy and happy longer.

PREVENTION is key!

If you gain just one piece of useful knowledge from my book to help you reach your health and wellness goals faster, then I'm one happy girl! And don't be afraid to let me know your thoughts afterwards, I'm all eyes!

Shall we...

Chapter One - What is Fat?

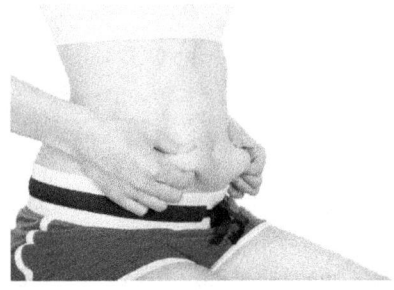

Simply put, fat is a macronutrient critical for normal body function, according to *Medical News Today.*

Without fat you couldn't survive. Fat provides readily available energy and makes it possible for your body to absorb and utilize other essential nutrients.

A Little Bit of Chemistry...

-Fats are large molecules of elements - Carbon, Hydrogen, and Oxygen
-The ratio of hydrogen to oxygen is 2-1
-Fats are insoluble molecules
-Fats are great molecules for storing - excess sugar intake is converted to fat
-The majority of dietary fat is in form of triglycerides
-Triglycerides form when 3 fatty acids are adhered to glycerol
-Any fatty acids in animal products are saturated
-Any fatty acids in plant foods are unsaturated for the most part
-Waxes are large lipid molecules
-Steroids are fat soluble compounds

Both fats and oils have two components...

FATTY ACIDS - These are long chains with just hydrogen and carbon in a chain. At the end of each chain there's a carboxyl group, -COOH.

GLYCEROL - This is a molecule with a hydroxyl group and 3 carbons. This 3 carbon molecule is the base of a fat molecule, according to *Odeca.*

BOTTOM LINE - YOU NEED FAT!

You're going to find fat in just about every food on the planet. There are even minute amounts in low-fat fruits and veggies.

Avocado - 35 calories fat per fruit, or 4.5 grams
Kiwi - 10 calories fat per fruit, or 1 gram

Peach - .5 grams fat per fruit

Sweet corn - 20 calories fat per cob, 2.5 grams

Broccoli - .5 grams of fat per cup

NOTE: These are healthy fats your body requires for optimal health. So the minute traces of fat in fruits and veggies is nothing to worry about.

Fat comes with different labels. Here are fats and their meanings.

Fats - This refers to all types of fat. Take note fats solid at room temperature are often called "fat."

Lipids - This is a universal term for fat whether the fat is liquid or solid.

Animal Fats - These are fats that are lard, cream, butter, or the fat naturally found in meat.

Oils - These are fats that are liquid at room temperature. They have a greasy feel and don't mix with water.

Veggie Fats - Examples are peanut oil, sunflower oil, corn oil, and olive oil.

If you eat too much fat, regardless of the type, you'll become obese. In fact, any nutrient you eat in excess, particularly unhealthy simple carbohydrates, will make you fat.

How much fat do you need?

Unfortunately there isn't an exact answer for this one. And according to *Penn Medicine,* most people don't have to worry about not getting enough fat in their diets.

Step One

Figure out how many calories your body expends at rest. This is also known as your BMI. This formula takes into consideration your sex, age, size, and level of activity. Understand your calorie needs are also reflective of your medical status, genetics, and specific nutrition goals.

The BMI calculator is a great place to start. It will give you a number to start with. This calculator is readily available online, or you can ask your doctor or nutritionist.

Step Two

Use this chart to figure out approximately how many fat grams you need to consume each day for ultimate health. Again, this is a platform to build from, a solid place to start!

CALORIES	FAT
1200	40
1300	43
1400	47
1500	50
1600	53
1700	56
1800	60
1900	63
2000	65
2100	70
2200	73
2300	77
2400	80
2500	83
2600	87
2700	90
2800	93
2900	97
3000	100

So, if you know the number of calories your body needs each day to function, you can figure out the general amount of fat you'll need to eat. Seems simple enough. The confusion comes when figuring out what type of fat you should be eating and how you can get it.

The Heart and Stroke Foundation of America states, 25-35% of your calories should come from fat.

Good Fat Serving Sizes

*2-3 servings per day

*1 tbsp. soft margarine

*1 tsp veggie oil
*1 tbsp. mayo
*1 tbsp. full-fat salad dressing
*2 tbsp. low-fat dressing

Those serving sizes are in accordance with heart.org.

Note - According to *Dietary Guideline for American*, children aged 2-18 should get 30-35% of their daily calories from fat.

Let's look at types of fats now!

My Thoughts...

Fat is something most people love to hate. We need in order to survive. But if you get too much of it, they'll be serious health consequences. Understanding the basics of fat helps you make healthier food choices, each of which pushes you forward closer to your personal health and wellness goals.

Chapter Two - Fat Types

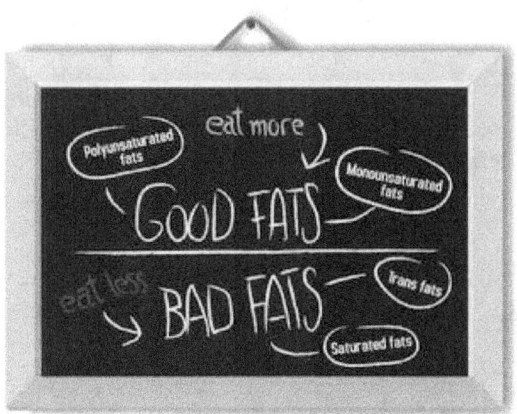

Most of us think of unhealthy (saturated) fat, and healthy (unsaturated) fat, when considering what kind of fat to eat.

However these two kinds of fat can be broken down further to make FOUR main types of fat.

Healthy Unsaturated Fat:

Monounsaturated fat
Polyunsaturated fat
-Omega-3 and 6 fat

Unhealthy Saturated Fat:

Saturated fat
Trans fat

Each of these fats reacts differently in your body. Some fat types help strengthen internal systems. Others, like synthetic trans fat, cause serious disease.

THE KEY - Understanding the characteristics of these fats, which to avoid, and what healthy fats you need in your diet and in what amounts.

UNSATURATED FAT - is a fatty acid that has one or more double bonds in the fatty acid chain, according to *Science Daily*. It's liquid at room temperature.

The fat molecule is *monounsaturated* if it's got a double bond, and *polyunsaturated* if it's got more than one double bond.

Interesting Fact - Hydrogen atoms are removed when double bonds are created. So saturated fat is loaded with hydrogen atoms.

*The more double bonds and less hydrogen atoms a fat has, the more volatile it is, and the quicker it goes bad. Antioxidants help protect volatile unsaturated healthy fat from going rancid.

Common Unsaturated Fat Foods

Monounsaturated Fat

*Avocado
*Nuts
*Seeds
*Peanut oil
*Olives and olive oil
*Canola oil
*Non-hydrogenated margarines

Polyunsaturated Fat

*Omega-6 - corn, sunflower, sesame, and corn oil, nuts, seeds, non-hydrogenated margarine

*Omega-3 - fattier fish, soybean oil, flax seed, walnuts, eggs with omega-3

SATURATED FAT - Are simply fat molecules that don't have any double bonds between carbon bonds, simply because they're saturated with hydrogen molecules. Most saturated fats are in a solid state at room temperature.

These fats are often found in processed fast foods, and packaged baked goods and pastries. They raise bad LDL cholesterol, which increases your risk of cardiovascular disease and stroke.

Natural Saturated Fat Found in Dairy Products:

*Chicken and other poultry with skin
*Beef
*Butter and cream
*Lard
*Cheese
*High-fat yogurt
*High-fat cottage cheese
*Whole milk

CIP - Cathy's Important Point - Various oils that are plant-based have saturated fat, but are void of cholesterol. Like coconut oil and palm oil.

Trans Fat - Minute amounts of this fat is naturally present in animal products. Although the majority of trans fat is synthetic. Made by adding hydrogen to veggie oil, and making it solid at room temperature.

Why is Dangerous trans fat used?

*Cheap for manufacturers
*Foods last longer on the shelf cuz molecules are more stable
*Makes food look and taste better

Note - A restaurant can fry with the same oil forever!

Trans Fat Foods

Snack Food - *Microwave popcorn, corn chips, potato chips, and tortilla chips.*

Baked Goods - *Cookies, cakes, pie crusts, crackers, frosting, and pastries.*

Fried Food - *French fries, donuts, fried chicken, and ribs.*

Refrigerator Dough - *Biscuits, cinnamon rolls, cookie batter, and frozen pizza.*

Creams/Margarines - *Stick margarine and nondairy coffee cream*

NOTE: The food labels in America are very misleading. A food that has .5 grams of fat in a serving can be labelled 0 grams of trans fat. A hidden bad fat that adds up quickly. Be wary just because the package says 0 grams of trans fat doesn't necessarily mean that.

My Thoughts...

Science says you can't survive without fat. You need it to think straight and function. It protects your internal organs, keeps you warm, and helps support smooth immune system function by assisting in vitamin absorption.

The problem stems from the type of fat you eat and in what quantities. 2-3 servings of healthy fat is all you need each day to be on top of your game. Time to focus on the BIG PICTURE of good health.

Chapter Three - Fat Facts

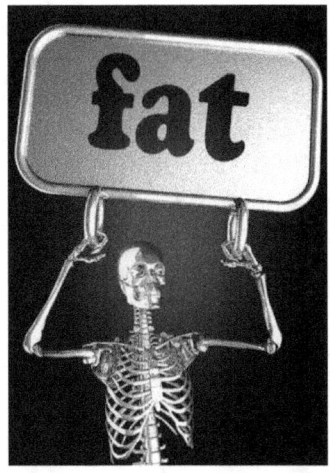

Gone are the days where people were taught to be afraid of fat. I remember my grandfather always telling me that fat would make me fat! Lovingly I say that's hogwash! Everybody needs fat. The tough part is sorting through the crap to get to the facts!

Here are a few facts you can take to beach!

FAT FACTS GOOD, BAD, AND DOWNRIGHT UGLY!

ONE -Fat supplies essential fatty-acids your body can't make, according to profession of nutrition *Wahida Karmally*.

TWO - Fat makes the absorption of fat soluble vitamins A, D, E, and K possible!

THREE - Fat has nine calories per gram. That's twice the calories the other two macronutrients, protein and carbs, have.

FOUR - According to *The Heart and Stroke Foundation of Canada*, saturated trans fat, or bad fat, is associated with cardiovascular disease and stroke.

FIVE - Too much bad fat increases bad cholesterol, clogging arteries and making your heart work stronger.

SIX - *The American Heart and Stroke Foundation* recommends 25 - 35% of your daily calories should come from good fat!

SEVEN - Good fats are found in...

*Olive, canola, sunflower and sesame oil
*Olives
*Avocado and nuts
*Sunflower and flax seed
*Soybeans
*Salmon and other seafood
*Healthy tub margarine

EIGHT - Omega fatty acids often found in fatty fish are imperative for the brain, heart, and eyesight development of children in particular.

NINE - Omega fats help reduce bad cholesterol, and improve blood flow to the brain, organs and body.

TEN - Saturated fat is found namely in fatty meat and natural dairy products. Highly saturated veggie fats like palm oil and cocoa butter are also very unhealthy. These are used in those yummy guilty pleasures like processed cookies, cakes, pastries, and crackers.

ELEVEN - Synthetic trans fat is more dangerous than unhealthy saturated fat to excess, and is linked to cancers, heart attacks, and oodles of deaths.

TWELVE - Trans fat is naturally found in microscopic amounts in animal products. Some experts believe when eaten naturally with a moderated low-fat diet, it actually helps deter disease. Problem is, people just have to be extreme!

THIRTEEN - Saturated fats are normally solid at room temperature.

FOURTEEN - According to a research study at Laval University, thinking hard can actually trigger fat gain. Too much thought triggers hunger, which encourages overeating and fat gain.

FIFTEEN - The average person has over fifty billion fat cells. That's more than the earth's population!

SIXTEEN - You don't grow new fat cells. They just get bigger or smaller depending on what you're eating and your caloric expenditure.

SEVENTEEN - Boobs are made of fat. Which explains why when I was pregnant I shifted from B cup to a full C. And since I've lost weight since having kids and kept it off for years, I'm sad to say I am now an A! Why can't breasts be made of all muscle??? :)

EIGHTEEN - You can't lose fat in one place, according to the experts at *Weightlossresources* in the UK. If you could, people that chew gum would have skinny faces!

NINETEEN - Alcohol has 7 calories per gram. Fat has 9 calories per gram. Protein and carbs have just 4 calories per gram.

TWENTY - Experts say fat cells live about ten years before they're replaced. However, brain cells die and aren't replaced. Which is why brain exercises are essential to preventing memory loss!

CIP - Cathy's Important Point - Truly Bizarre - I don't think you're going to argue with *Women's Day* about the fact *The Tapeworm Diet*, is one of the dumbest diets ever!

This is where people would knowingly eat baby tapeworms so these worms will eat all the food in their intestines, and help people lose weight! OMG! Apart from eating disgusting worms, you've also got to consider the facts these worms can grow to TWENTY-FIVE feet, and cause seizures, dementia, and meningitis. YIKES!

I'm good with just eating healthy and exercising regularly thank-you!

My Thoughts...

There's always something to learn about fat. Cuz the more information you have, the better the decisions you'll make to take you straight to your health and wellness goals. Hope you learned a few things that'll help you create your master health plan for life.

Chapter Four - Fat Benefits

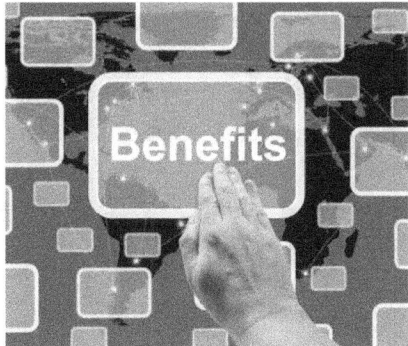

We've been talking about fat now for three chapters. I've put together a list of fat benefits just to reiterate the cold hard fact, you NEED healthy fat for optimal health. You also need to eat fat in moderation to lose weight.

Proven Benefits of Fat

INCREASED MUSCLE

Having healthy amounts of fat on your body encourages balance, and the optimal environment for healthy lean muscle growth. Fat helps you recover from intense exercising faster, while elevating growth hormone, which deters muscle breakdown, IF you're also restricting carbs.

Healthy fat will give you a tighter body.

LESS RESISTANCE TO WEIGHT LOSS

If you don't eat enough fat calories to sustain body function, you'll communicate to your body to shut down. You're not providing your body with the energy to function, sending it into "starvation mode." Everything you eat will be stored as fat. Your energy levels will be low, and your metabolism will slow. Which of course makes it extremely difficult to lose weight.

Bottom line is, you've gotta feed your body enough good fat to WANT to burn fat for fuel. Eat healthy fat in moderation to lose weight and you will!

IMPROVES BODY COMPOSITION

According to *Poliquingroup,* you need fat to stay lean because...

*Fat makes up the outer most layer of your cells. This layer makes your body sensitive to insulin resistance, reduces inflammation, and encourages energy for metabolism.

*Eating Omega fats flips to switch for the fat burning process.

*Fat fills you up, encouraging you to feel satisfied with less, and eat less because of this!

*Cholesterol comes from fat and encourages normal hormone balance. You're going to lose weight faster with a better hormone balance.

Fat increases metabolism, balances hormones, and reduces sugary fatty cravings!

BETTER MOOD AND THOUGHT FUNCTION

Your noggin is made of fat and cholesterol. The majority should be DHA, an essential fatty acid. The fat in your brain

28

influences all the electrical nerve impulses, dictating everything from hormone levels and mood, to clear thinking and energy. Having enough healthy fat in your regular diet deters depression, and decreases serotonin, your natural "feel good" chemical.

For clear thinking and optimal brain function you need to ensure you get healthy fat daily, this includes your omega-3s at least twice a week!

INCREASES CHANCE OF GETTING PREGNANT

I know through personal experience, if a woman doesn't have enough healthy body fat, her body will stop ovulating. If there is no ovulation or release of an egg or ovum, fertilization can't occur, and this means no baby.

Menstruation monthly is a signal that fat stores are adequate and reproduction may occur. Although even when a woman menstruates, this doesn't mean she's ovulated. Three are specific symptoms you can look for to verify ovulation. Like egg white cervical mucus, increased sex drive, high ripe cervix, and even ovulation pain or slight bleeding when the egg is released. A rise is basil body temperature can verify after-the-fact that ovulation has occurred.

Fat helps ensure the natural process of reproduction can occur.

DECREASED RISK OF OSTEOPOROSIS

Woman's Day states that fats are necessary for calcium metabolism, and fat-soluble vitamins K and D are essential to build strong bones.

LOWERS RISK OF CANCER AND CARDIOVASCULAR DISEASE

Inflammation has been observed as a trigger for cancer. Good fats reduce this risk. Studies show healthy monounsaturated fat, like olive oil, help prevent cancer.

IMPROVED SKIN HEALTH

If you've got dry eyes, you may be lacking healthy fatty acids. Ensuring you get at least 3 g of omega-3s each day, combined with a variety of healthy fats, will improve your skin health.

STRONGER IMMUNE SYSTEM FUNCTION

Coconut oil is the one saturated fat that's an exception to the rules. There are oodles of health benefits both in food and topical. Everything from clearing minor skill ailments and conditioning skin, to fighting fungal infections and improving internal immune system function.

Just remember when cooking with coconut oil, to use it in moderation. Too much of anything isn't a good thing!

My Thoughts...

The benefits of fat in your diet are crystal clear. In moderation fat is essential to your good health. For most of us it's important to make sure we are eating healthy fat in moderation. 2-3 servings is all you need each day. Too much of any fat will make you fat!

Chapter Five - Fat and Disease

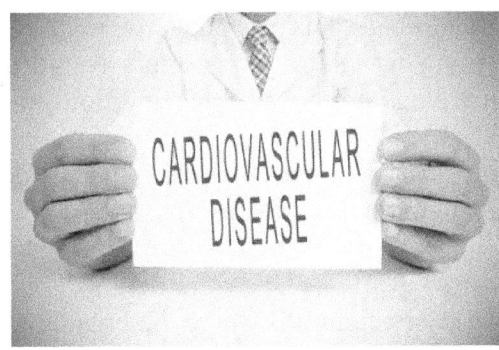

According to *WebMD* there are numerous diseases linked to fat, or obesity. If you weigh twenty percent more than your ideal weight, that's considered obese. Where your risk for serious disease increases.

Centers for Disease Control and Prevention, says over **one-third** of Americans are obese!

Main Diseases Associated With Fat

*Cardiovascular Disease and Stroke - When you're carrying extra fat, you naturally increase the risk of elevated blood pressure and cholesterol. Both of which boost your risk for stroke and heart disease.

Fitness experts at **_shape.com_** say, by losing just ten percent of your body weight, the odds of developing these issues decreases drastically.

*Various Cancers - Breast, colon, kidney, reproductive, and throat cancers are all associated with fat.

*Elevated Blood Pressure

*Arthritis - Joint conditions often develop in fat people. The natural cushioning around the joints wears away from all excess weight, causing various arthritic conditions to develop.

*Gout - If you have too much uric acid in your blood, a joint condition called gout may develop.

*Sleep Troubles - Apnea - This condition is directly linked to people that are overweight. It's where the breathing passage is blocked or constricted, often because of neck fat, and the breathing stops up to 50 times an hour in serious cases. This stresses the heart and internal systems, and affects normal function the next day.

*Asthma - Another respiratory issue often associated with overweight people.

*Type 2 Diabetes - The majority of people with type two or adult onset diabetes are overweight. Some people with this condition can lose weight and control their glucose levels naturally. Others will need to take insulin to control their blood sugar levels.

*Gallbladder Disease - When you're overweight, gallstones and gallbladder disease are more likely. Make note that if you drop fat too quickly, you increase the likelihood of developing gallstones. Experts recommend 1-2 pounds per week is the safest and most permanent rate to lose weight.

*If fat happens to gather around your middle, your risk of developing many diseases increases.

My Thoughts...

Prevention is the focus. By taking control of your health by eating right and exercising, you'll naturally lose weight and decrease the risk of developing fat-related diseases. This doesn't mean you won't ever face them. But working hard to keep your weight within the normal range will lower your odds significantly.

It's a matter of choice...

Chapter Six - Fat Foods

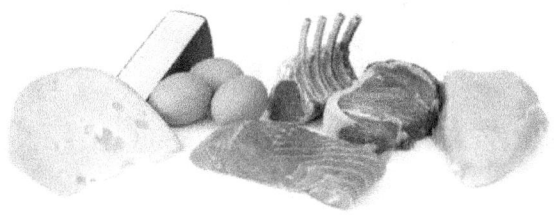

There's a gynormous difference between good and bad fat foods. However, ultimately it's the total number of calories you consume that determines whether or not you've got extra padding.

I'm going to break this down into healthy fat foods and unhealthy. For the most part you should always opt for the good stuff, in moderation of course!

Healthy Fatty Foods

*Beef - Unfortunately when it comes to eating meat, most people opt for chicken or fish because it's considered lean. This means beef often gets left out, because people think of it as a bad fat meat.

This is partially correct. If you're looking to lose weight and lower your overall fat intake, choosing the lowest fat meats is a wise-owl move. But this doesn't mean beef with higher fat is all bad.

Here are a few reasons the saturated fat in beef isn't so bad:

1- Almost half the fat found in beef is oleic acid, or monoun-saturated. This is heart healthy fat you'll find in olives.

2- According to *Men's Health*, the majority of saturated fat found in beef lowers the risk of cardiovascular disease. This happens by either lowering LDL or bad cholesterol, or shrinking the ratio between good cholesterol and total cholesterol.

Nutrition - 1 cup of shredded beef has about 350 calories, 15 grams fat, and 32 grams of protein.

Add to this all the essential vitamins and minerals found in meat, and you'll see you should embrace beef in moderation, don't run from it.

Eggs - Eggs not only contain the most vitamins and minerals per ounce, they've got choline, something your body needs to breakdown fat.

Studies at Saint Louis University found people that ate eggs instead of simple carb bagels, consumed less calories the rest of the day.

Gone are the day's experts preached eggs are dangerous for the heart and cholesterol levels. In moderation, eggs will do your body fantabulous!

Nutrition - 1 egg has about 70 calories, 5 grams of fat, and just over 6 grams of protein.

Cheese - Hard cheese is packed with protein and fat, to help calm your hunger by giving you that full feeling. It's also dense in calories, so a little goes along way. Cheese is also extremely versatile, and a little goes a long way!

Nutrition - 1 ounce or 28 grams of cheddar has 110 calories, 10 grams of fat, and about 7 grams of protein.

Coconut - Maybe we should call it controversial coconut? Coconut technically has more saturated fat than butter.
BUT...experts believe it's heart healthy, according to *Shape* magazine.

Why?

Research studies from the *American Journal of Clinical Nutrition,* states more than half the saturated fat is lauric acid, which lowers your risk of cardiovascular disease by decreasing bad cholesterol and raising good.

Furthermore, the remaining saturated fat doesn't seem to negatively affect cholesterol levels.

Nutrition - 1 piece of raw coconut, or about 45 grams, has 150 calories, 15 grams of fat, 1.5 grams of protein, and 4 grams of fiber.

Avocado - Otherwise known as "butter pears," avocados are mainly fat, but it's healthy monounsaturated fat. Deemed to lower nasty LDL cholesterol and support heart health.

In fact, according to ***self.com***, the US government is officially encouraging Americans to eat more avocados.

Moderation is key.

Nutrition - 1/2 an avocado, 2 ounces, or about 60 grams, has nearly 2 grams of fiber, 100 calories, and 9 grams of fat.

Nuts - *Livescience* reports people that eat nuts are normally thinner, less likely to develop diabetes, and reduce the risk of heart disease. Almonds for instance, give you a taste of 17 vitamin and minerals!

Go for salt-free and keep it in moderation, because even though nuts are loaded with healthy fat, it's still fat.

Nutrition - About an ounce of almonds has almost 200 calories, 7 grams of protein, and about 16 grams of fat.

Fatty Fish - According to experts at **_self.com_**, fatty or oily fish like sardines, tuna, and salmon, are loaded with healthy omega-3 fatty acids. *The American Heart Association* states, you should enjoy at least a couple servings of these heart-healthy fats each week!

Nutrition - A 3-4 ounce serving of wild salmon has about 350 calories, 22 grams of healthy fat, 39 grams of muscle building protein, and zero carbs.

Unhealthy Fatty Foods

Since there are so many unhealthy fat foods, I'm going to list them a little differently. Not so technical and tedious for you to read, and so we can cover more ground. I could give you all the nutritional info of chocolate chip cookies, oatmeal cookies, ginger cookies, raspberry muffins, banana muffins, etc. Problem is, there's too many different varieties and the message is still the same.

STAY CLEAR OF THESE TYPES OF FOOD WHEN YOU CAN!

SATURATED FAT AND TRANS FAT

*Convenient Fast Food

Most people use fast food eating as their daily staple because it's convenient and often cost affective. It's only a buck or two for a grease burger. FFF suppresses hunger fast, and plants an addictive seed in your brain to want more.

VERY POWERFUL!

Fast food options are typically very high in calories, with little nutrition and oodles of bad fat, often trans fat.

Greasy double burgers with cheese, fries, shakes, chicken nuggets, chicken wings, and poutine, are all LOADED with crap.

We eat them because we can, not because our intrinsic body says we should, in order to function optimally!

These fast foods clog arteries, make your heart work harder, trigger obesity, lead to diabetes, steal energy, send your blood glucose levels on a roller coaster, trigger mood swings, and leave you feeling like a blob of crap!

One burger gives you 40% of your daily sodium intake, and about 25% of your total caloric intake for the average woman. Are you freaking kidding me?

*Packaged Cookies

DON'T FORGET! Just because a product is labeled "Trans Fat Free," doesn't mean it's the case! Nutrition guidelines state if a food has .5% or less trans fat, it can be labelled free of this fat. To me that's a cheap and misleading move. Cuz .5+.5+.5+.5 = 2, and that's 2 grams too much of trans fat!

Here are a few packaged cookies to steer clear of...

Pepperidge Farm Chocolate Chip Brand - Smaller cookie, about 50 calories per soft cookie

Entenmann's Brand - These are mini cookies so you're more likely to go overboard, with 50 calories per cookie.

Chips Ahoy - A handful of 3 cookies is a whopping 160 calories, and 4 grams fat

Keebler Deluxe - These have 80 freakin calories per cookie!

Oreo's - Just 3 has about 170 calories and 7 grams of fat.

According to nutrition data at *Self*, most packaged cookies have at least 150 calories per 2-3 cookie serving, with about 6 grams of fat.

Cake and Pastry Frosting

Many people forget about this one because it's thought of as an add-on. Just a little something extra on your cake or Danish. Unless you're making your frosting carefully from scratch, you're likely to be heading into trans fat territory with icing in general. Duncan Hines Chocolate Frosting has enough trans fat to overload you for the day.

Your wise-owl move is to skip the frosting. Better yet, read the nutrition label and see for yourself. Or you could always get grandma to make you some the old-fashioned way. Even then you're still giving your body something it doesn't need.

Pancakes and Biscuit Mix

Buying box mixes is nothing but trouble in the fat department. In a cup of *Bisquick*, you're getting about FIVE grams of trans fat, according to bembu.com.

Keep in mind that boxed food items last for centuries on the shelf because they are filled with preservatives and stable fat, which is both saturated and trans fat in nature.

Quick Fix Microwave Popcorn

In general, most microwave popcorn brands have trans fat somewhere. It's often hidden behind the fact many companies advertise low-fat or no-fat varieties. The only way to know for sure on this one is to read the label and reflect!

FANTABULOUS OPTION...Eat a bowl of sweet corn, or pop your own naked popcorn, and sprinkle with water and a little salt if you must!

Frozen Entrees

These convenient frozen meals are often loaded with hydrogenated oils. This is a direct ticket to synthetic trans fat. Heating by microwaving also takes what's left of the nutrients out. There's no way around this one, but to cook your own meals from scratch, or read the label before you buy.

SATURATED FAT AND HFCS (HIGH FRUCTOSE CORN SYRUP) FOODS

HFCS was created until the 60s. It's used because it's very sweet, cheap to make, and it stores nicely. This fake sweetener often found in bad fat foods isn't programed into your body. There's no shut-off switch the way you can turn off natural simple sugars found in fruits for example.

Addictive and sweet are two lethal combinations. Triggering overeating, obesity, and oodles of diseases.

Pop or Soda

Soda manufacturers abundantly use HFCS to sweeten the beverage. Have a look for yourself! *Women's Day* states *Coca-Cola* uses high fructose corn syrup as the only sweetener.

CIP - Cathy's Important Point - According to *USA Today*, Pepsi plans on launching 3 varieties of Pepsi made with real sugar instead of HFCS. Ra-ra for them! This still can't negate the fact one can of Soda has a whopping 41 grams of sugar and 150 calories. Never mind the "type" of sweetener used, cuz it's WAY too much regardless!

Condiments - BBQ Sauce, Ketchup

The 3rd place ingredient on a bottle of ketchup is HFCS. Most of the sweetness in ketchup comes from this addictive stuff.

Sweetened Cereals

People have been programmed to think all cereals are a healthy start to the day. Problem is, many of the brand names, including *Kellogg's*, loads the favorites up with high fructose corn syrup to sweeten. It's cheap and addictive, a food manufacturer's dream!

Post and General Mills also do it. Make sure you read the ingredient list before you buy a box of *Lucky Charms* or *Frosted Flakes*!

My Thoughts...

Not all fat foods are detrimental to your good health. You need fat to lose fat, gain energy, and sustain good health. However, it's the kind of fat foods you're eating that determine whether or not you're setting yourself up for better health, or oodles of issues down the road.

PREVENTION is everything. Learning about the good, bad, and downright ugly of fat by reading my book, is your first step toward a healthier you!

Chapter Seven - Tips to Eat Healthy Fat

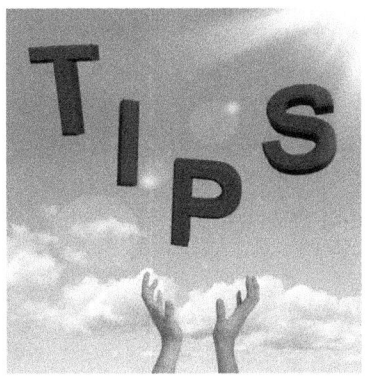

Small steps seems to be the way to go for most people when it comes to making healthier eating changes that stick. You and I are creatures of habit. And unless we consciously set up specific steps to make changes, and truly want to make these *specific* change, it's just not going to happen.

ACTION STEPS

*Decide to make a change

*Practice this change repeatedly

*Transform it into habit

*Get support

*Check in with yourself regularly to makes sure this new healthy habit sticks

*Continue reading my books to gain the knowledge and inspiration to make healthier changes (:))

*Rinse and repeat

Why Eat Less Fat Reminders...

*Helps you lose flubber

*Decreases the risk for serious disease like diabetes, stroke, and cardiovascular disease

*May lower your cancer risk

*Boosts energy

*Sharpens the noggin

*Makes room for healthy eating mentally and physically

Pointers to Help You Reduce Bad Fat and Eat Healthy Fat

*Eat your salad naked or have a dash of reduced or no-fat dressing.

*Ditch the high-fat extras like mayo and butter, for low-fat spreads like jam, or a thin layer of peanut butter. Even a dash of barbecue sauce or mustard is the lesser of the two evils when considering mayo or ranch sauce on your sandwich.

*Skip the sour cream on potatoes, and cheese on broccoli. Opt for herbs and spices instead, and save the fat and calories for another day.

*Flavor meats and pastas with herbs and spices, or tomato based sauce. It's better than rich creamy sauces, oils, and but-

ter. All that does is add a whopping number of fat calories to your dish you don't need!

*Switch from whole milk to skim. Do the same with yogurt, cottage cheese, and other dairy products.

*Watch your portion control! A 2x2 inch cube of cheese is a serving, 1/2 cup yogurt, 1 cup milk,1 slice whole grain bread, 1/2 sweet potato, 1-2 tbsp. salad dressing, 1 tablespoon peanut butter, 1/4 cup nuts, 3-4 ounces of meat, 1 cup veggies, 1 piece of fruit or 3/4 cup fruit cup, 1/2 cup cooked whole wheat pasta or rice, and 1/2 cup low-fat frozen yogurt, are all single servings.

*Stick with clean eating. This means eat foods that are as close to Mother Nature as possible.

*Cook your food healthier. This means choosing to steam, broil, bake, grill, and poach. Never mind the high-fat frying.

*Try not to add fat while cooking. This means use herbs and spices instead of butter or oil. You can also spray a pan with cooking spray, or put a drizzle of oil in the pan and wipe the excess out with a paper towel. This saves oodles of added calories in the long run.

*_Men's Health_ says deprivation usually backfires. If you really love dessert, try saving it for a special occasion. Or you can share it with a friend. Take 2-3 bites and set your fork down. It's a choice!

*When eating out, make sure you put half your dish in a doggy bag BEFORE you start eating! We train ourselves to finish everything on our plate. When we really should just eat until satisfied.

*Take small bites and chew your food slowly. Experts at <u>medi-cine.net</u> report findings where people that took the time to consciously chew their food, ate less food and lost more weight faster.

*Remove ALL junk food from cupboards, fridge, and your closet! At least if you get a craving for something fattening and it's not within reach, there's a little more time to think about what you really don't want to do!

*By adding 1/4 of an avocado, and handful of almonds, or a drizzle of olive oil to your salad, you're giving your body the healthy polyunsaturated omega-3 and omega-6 fatty acids it requires. These are heart healthy and lower cholesterol, according to <u>health.com</u>.

*_Newsflash_ - Less than ten percent of your total daily intake should come from saturated fat, says the _Dietary Guidelines for Americans_. So for every 1,000 calories, less than 11 grams should be from saturated fat. A 200 calorie serving of corn chips has 10 grams of fat. That's your maximum daily limit in one bang!

*Learning to read the label will do wonders when it comes to reducing fat. It won't take you long to understand the difference between unsaturated, saturated, and trans fats. This will help you make better food choices for you.

*Stick with clear soups, like chicken noodle and vegetable, instead of thick and creamy options, like cream or celery or broccoli, or French onion soup.

My Thoughts...

Learning to make better fat choices is an always and forever learning process. Keep your mind open to always gathering *new information about what foods you should and shouldn't be eating, and how much.*

Step by step you'll create new fat-friendly eating habits that your body and mind will thank you for!

Final Thoughts

Healthy Eating nutrition experts say you need fat. Fat gives you energy, helps you absorb essential fat soluble vitamins, protects internal organs, and helps maintain your internal body temperature. Good or unsaturated fat protects your heart, deter some cancers, and keeps your body healthy.

Saturated, trans fat, or bad fat triggers obesity, heart disease, stroke, diabetes, and a whole whack of other preventable diseases.

Critical Note - Making sure you are choosing healthy fat foods in moderation is critical to good health.

It's a matter of committing to positive health changes.

Wise-Owl Move - Out with the junk-food fat, and in with the healthy unsaturated fat in moderation.

These are your life decisions only YOU can make. By job is to use this book to introduce you to fat and the role it plays in your existence. Now it's up to you to take what works for you and run with it.

Every positive health change you turn into habit, makes you healthier than you were yesterday. And that's something to be proud of. Time for you to take action toward better health!

Last Thoughts…

*THANK-YOU for reading my masterpiece. I hope you learned a little something, or at least got a few smiles.
*I would appreciate a millisecond or three of your time for a quick review, to help me build my masterful book empire higher.
*Whatever you do, don't forget to smile, and of course, check out my website for more of my e-Book masterpieces at: www.flawlesscreativewriting.com

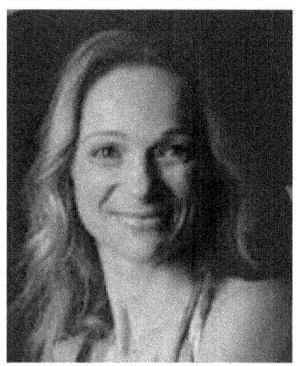

Thank you!
Cathy ☺